Eva the Hungry Amoeba

Goes on an Adventure
DNA & Cells

Eva the hungry amoeba introduces
young children to nutrients, in a fun
story where Eva learns which
foods to eat to help her grow

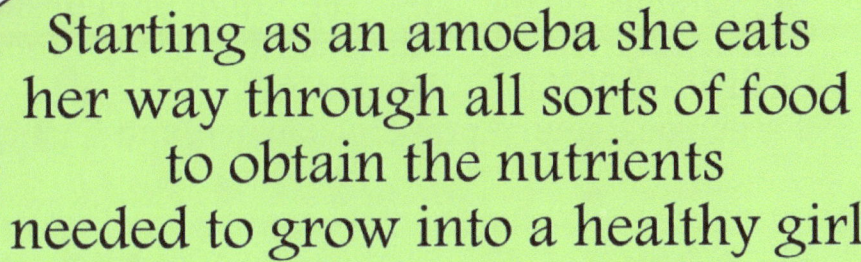

Starting as an amoeba she eats
her way through all sorts of food
to obtain the nutrients
needed to grow into a healthy girl

Published by Check Your Food Ltd
Brighton UK

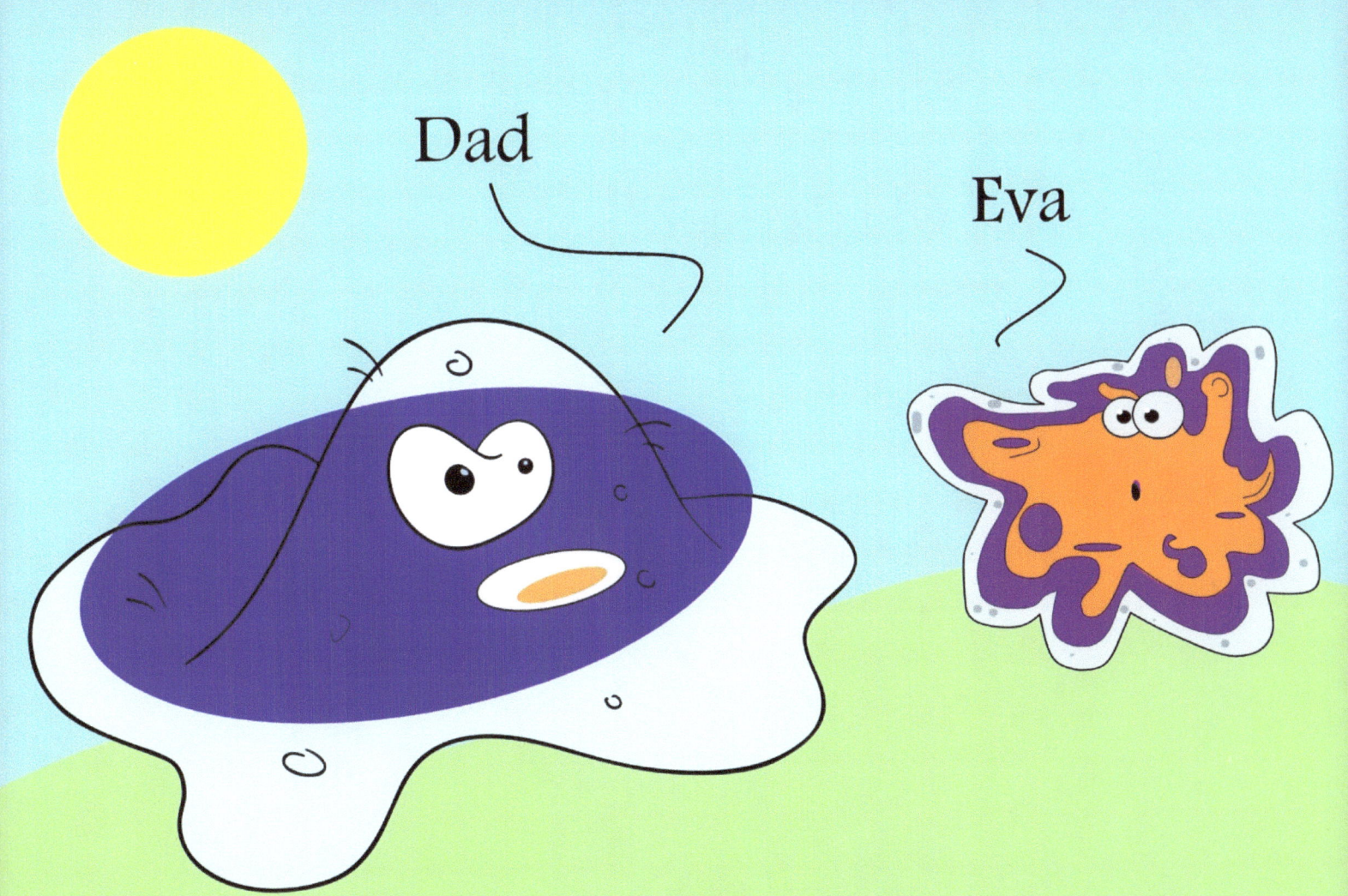

Meet Eva, the very, very, very hungry amoeba
She was so greedy, she ate everyone's food
"Eva" said dad "don't be so rude
Go on an adventure, now off you go
Eat the right food and maybe you'll grow"

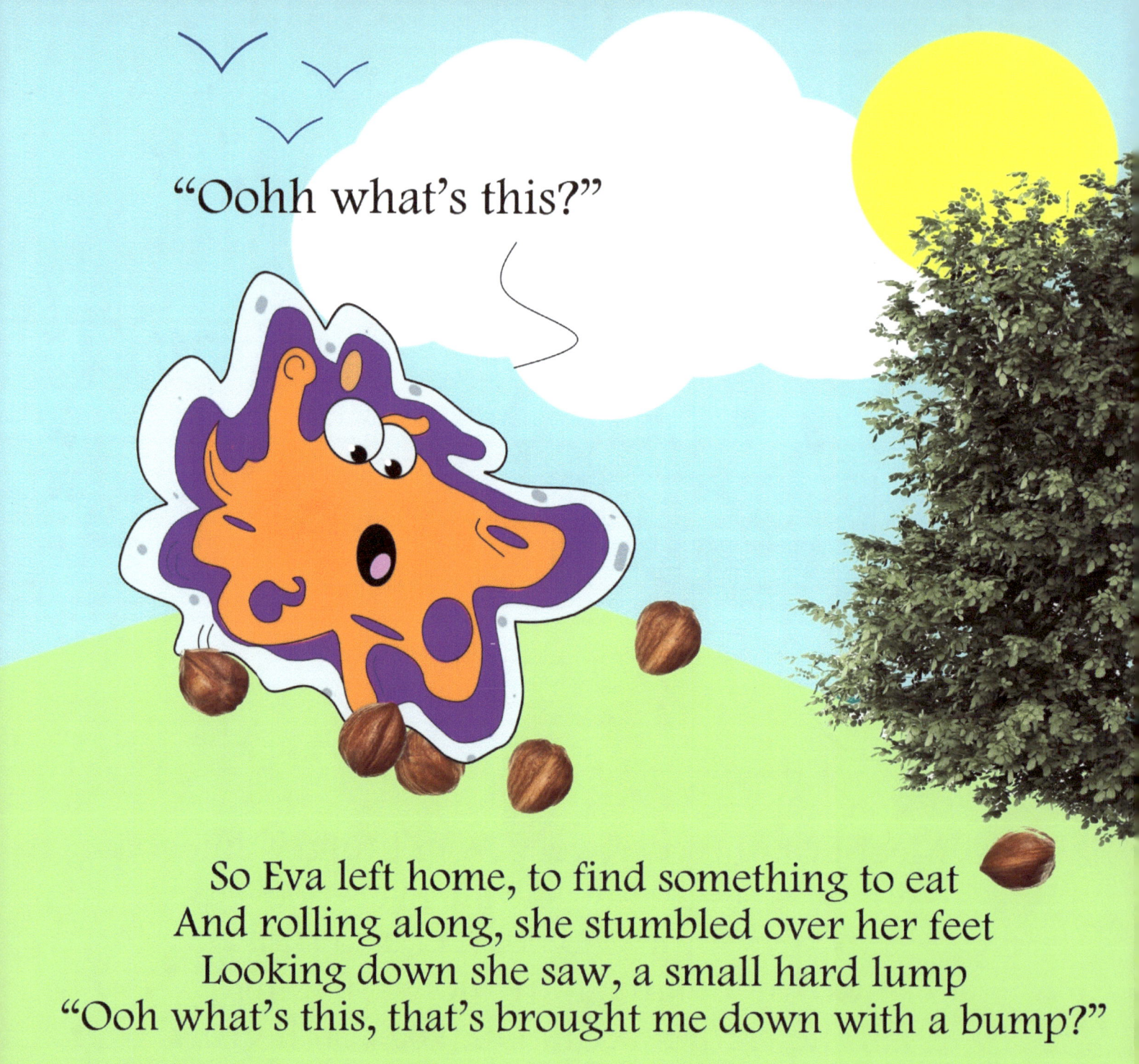

So Eva left home, to find something to eat
And rolling along, she stumbled over her feet
Looking down she saw, a small hard lump
"Ooh what's this, that's brought me down with a bump?"

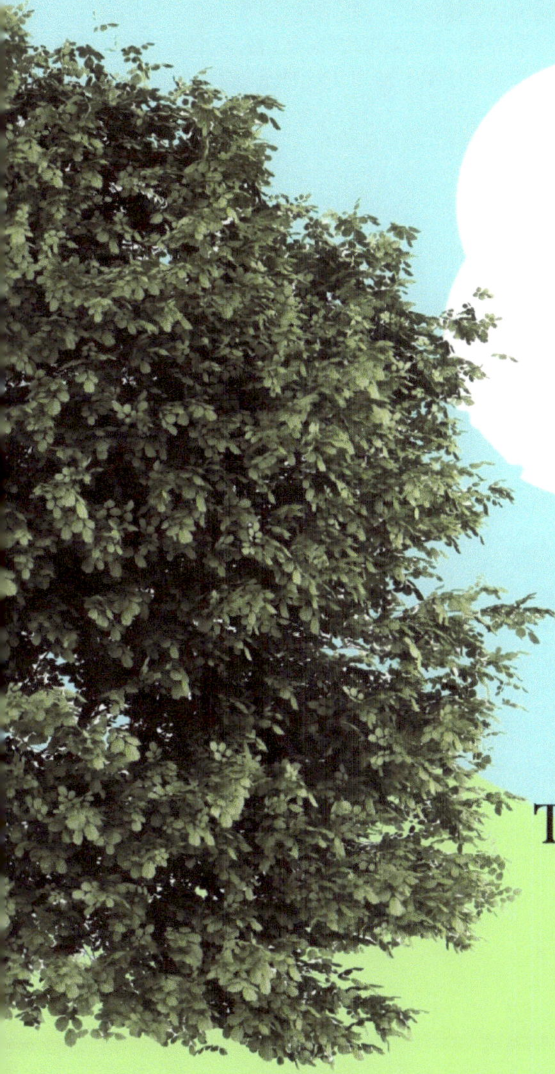

"And more importantly
Can I eat it for lunch?"

Enter the Hazelnut

Eva crunched it down
With biotin too
When her cells and
DNA shouted "woohoo"
They were starting to multiply
Which is a good thing
If you want to be able
To dance and sing

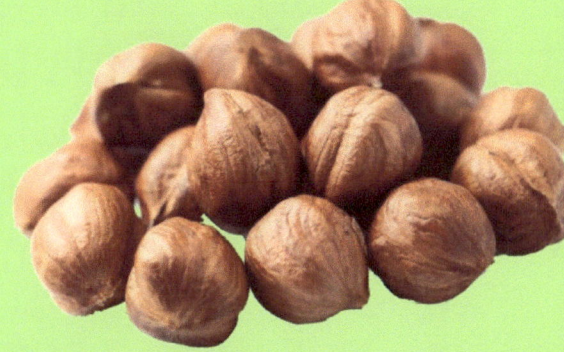

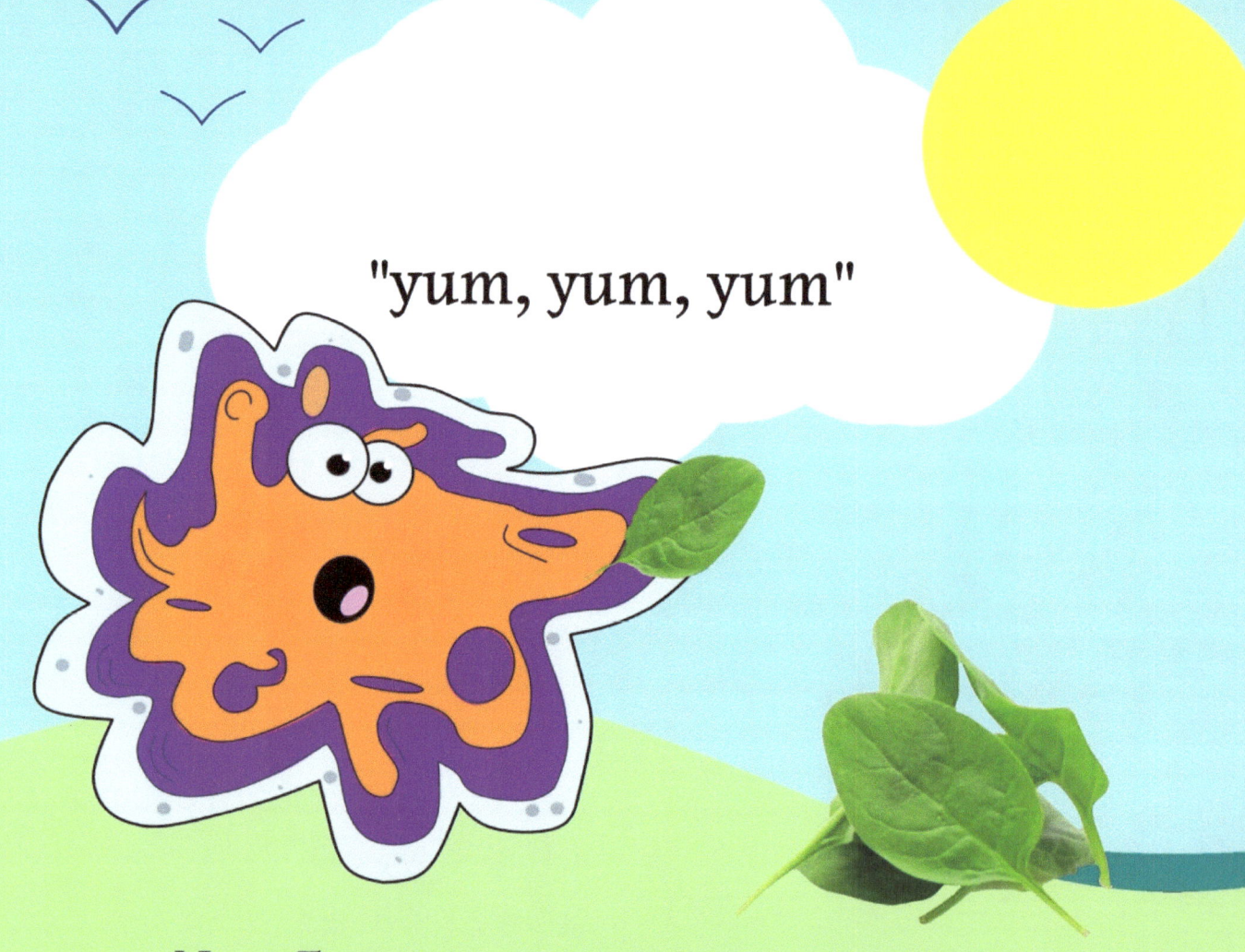

"yum, yum, yum"

Now Eva was even more ravenous
Her tummy was feeling rather cavernous
So off she set to find her next meal
But she was so hungry she started to reel
Not a moment too soon she saw something green
"Yum, yum, yum" she started to scream!

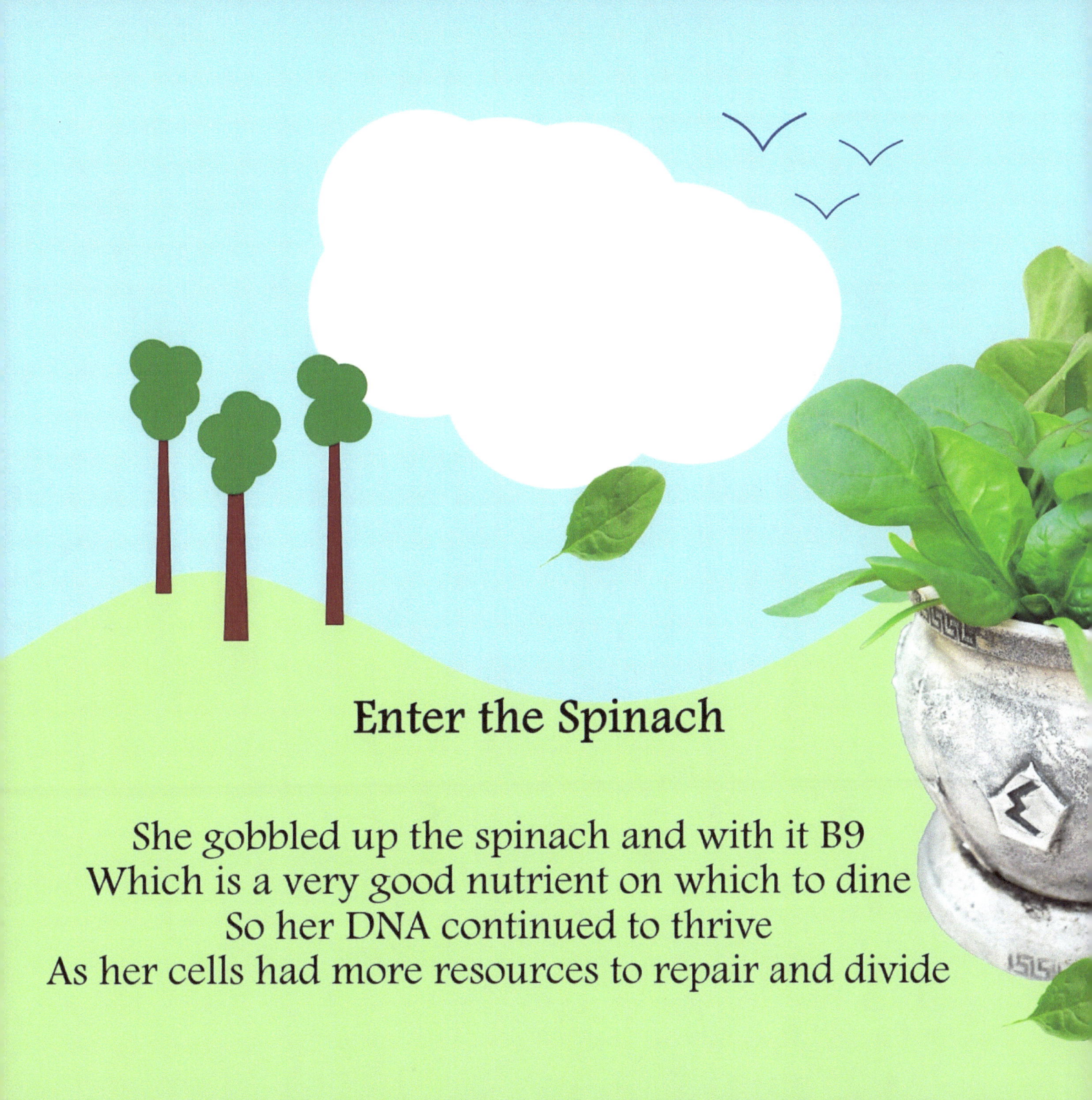

Enter the Spinach

She gobbled up the spinach and with it B9
Which is a very good nutrient on which to dine
So her DNA continued to thrive
As her cells had more resources to repair and divide

Inside Eva, her cells were moving
Dividing, multiplying, really grooving
There were blood cells
And fat cells
And nerve cells and more
All increasing to help Eva soar

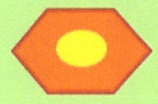

Liver cells

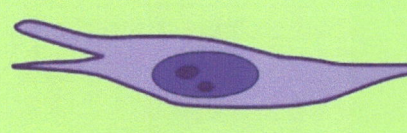

Skin cells

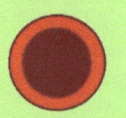

Blood cells

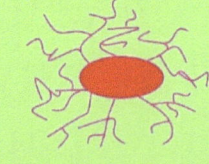

Nerve cells

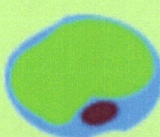

Fat cells

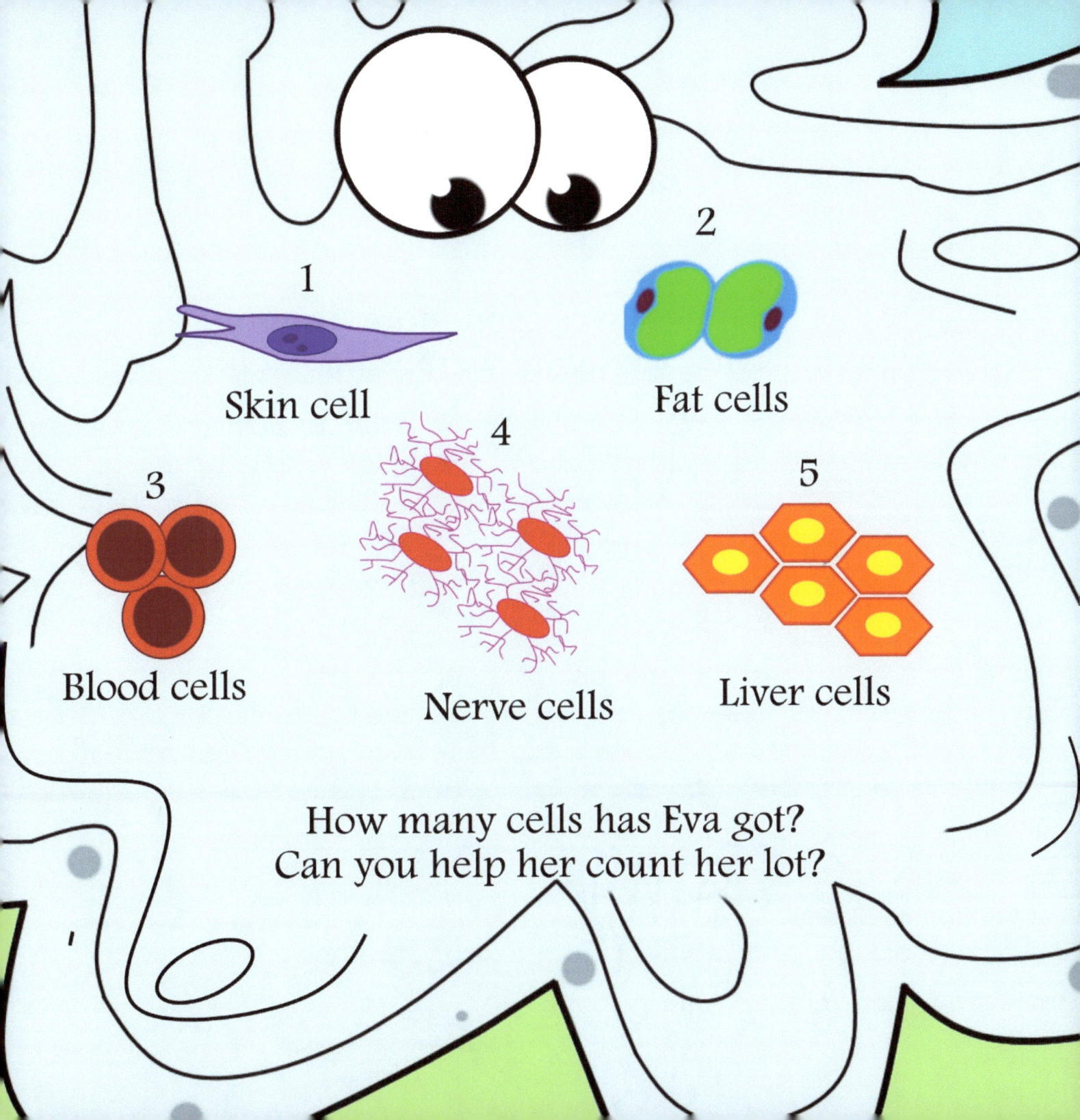

1 Skin cell

2 Fat cells

3 Blood cells

4 Nerve cells

5 Liver cells

How many cells has Eva got?
Can you help her count her lot?

Enter the Eggs

Eva, who now was even more hungry
Spotted some eggs who were rather funky
They were giggling and playing and having fun
Until one fell down on its fragile bum!

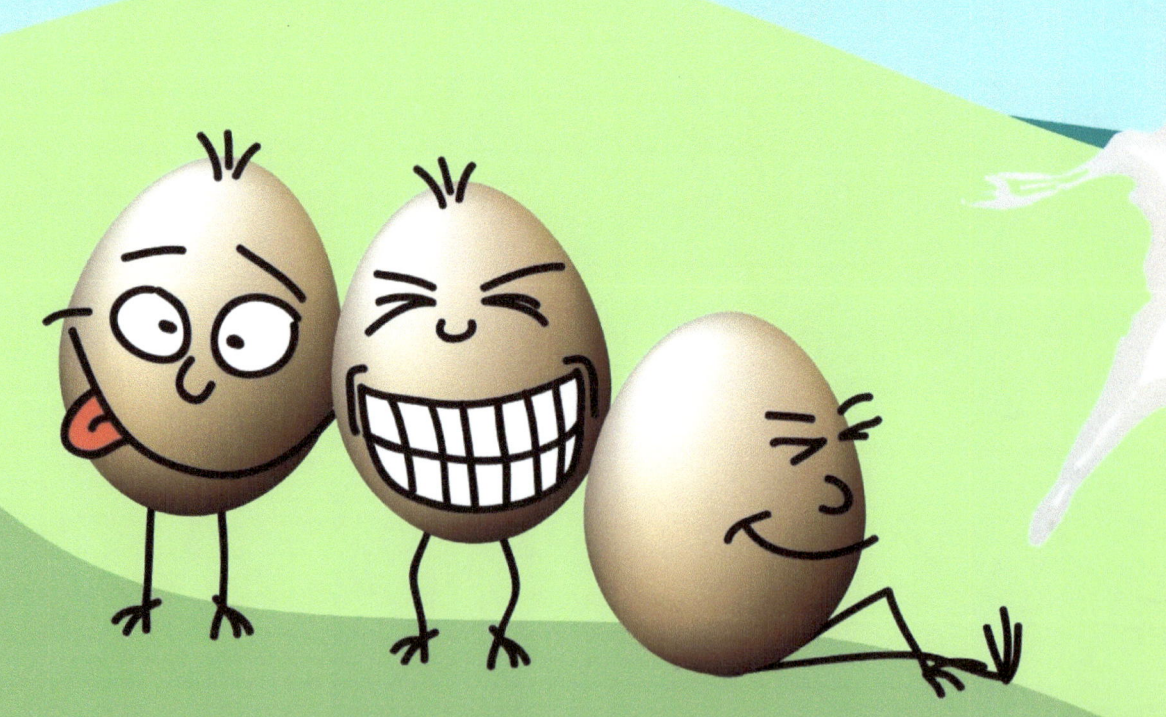

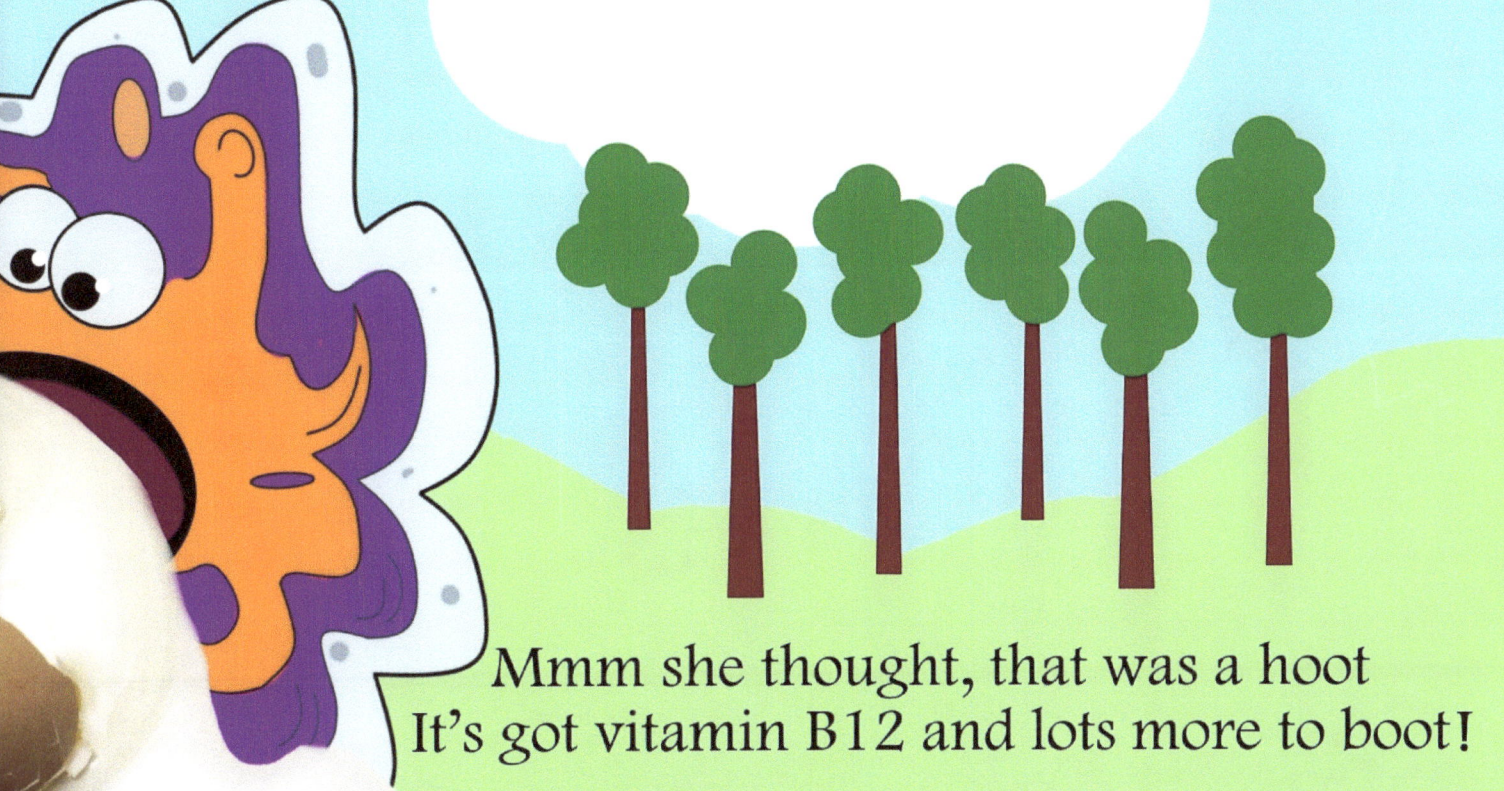

Splosh went the egg, all over the floor
Eva gobbled it up and went looking for more

Mmm she thought, that was a hoot
It's got vitamin B12 and lots more to boot!

Eggs are a fab ingredient, with which to nourish
A little amoeba, who wants to flourish

So Eva continued along her way
Looking for more food and a chance to play
When suddenly she sank up to her knees
In water full of spiky leaves

Enter the Rice

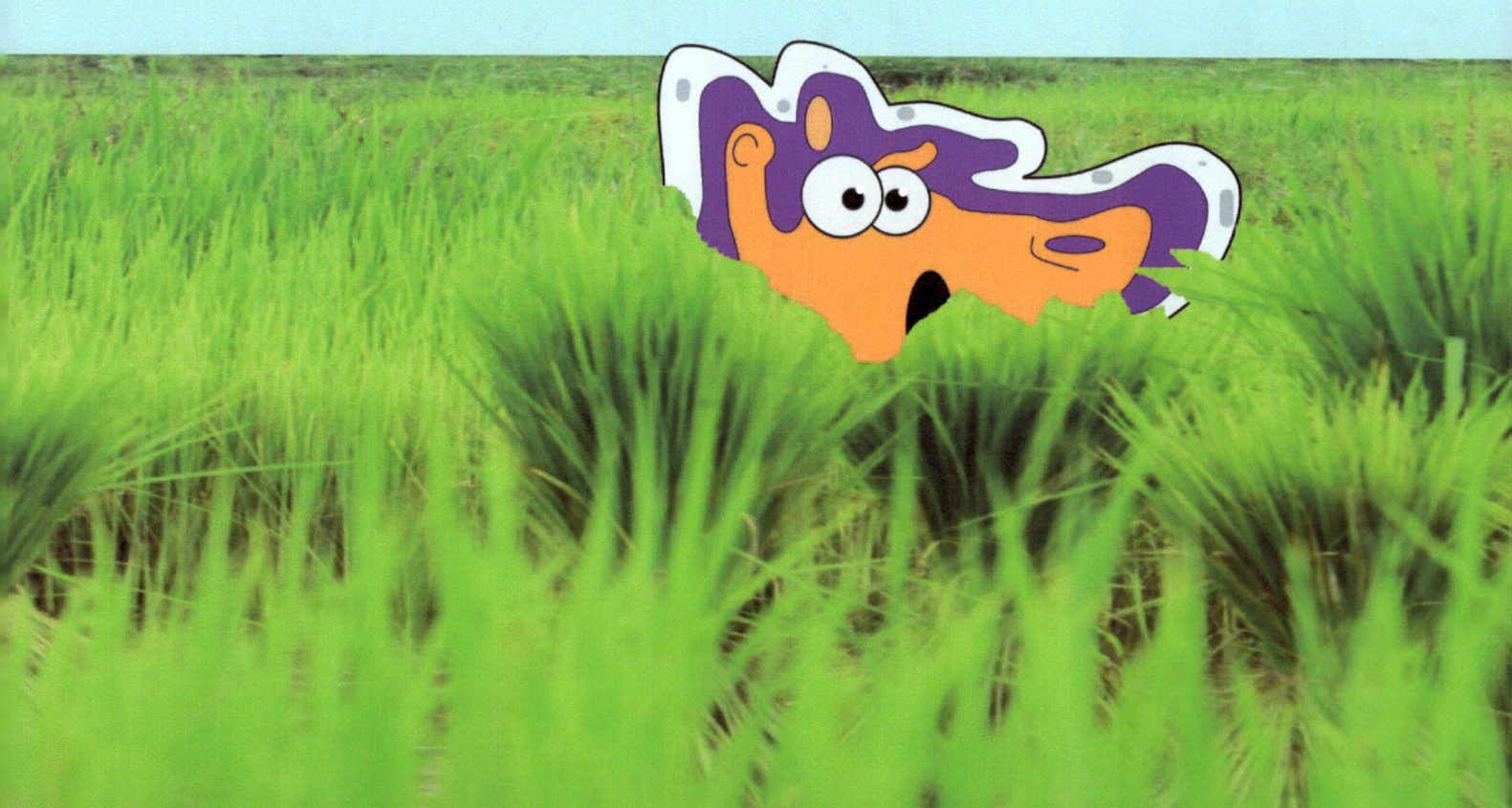

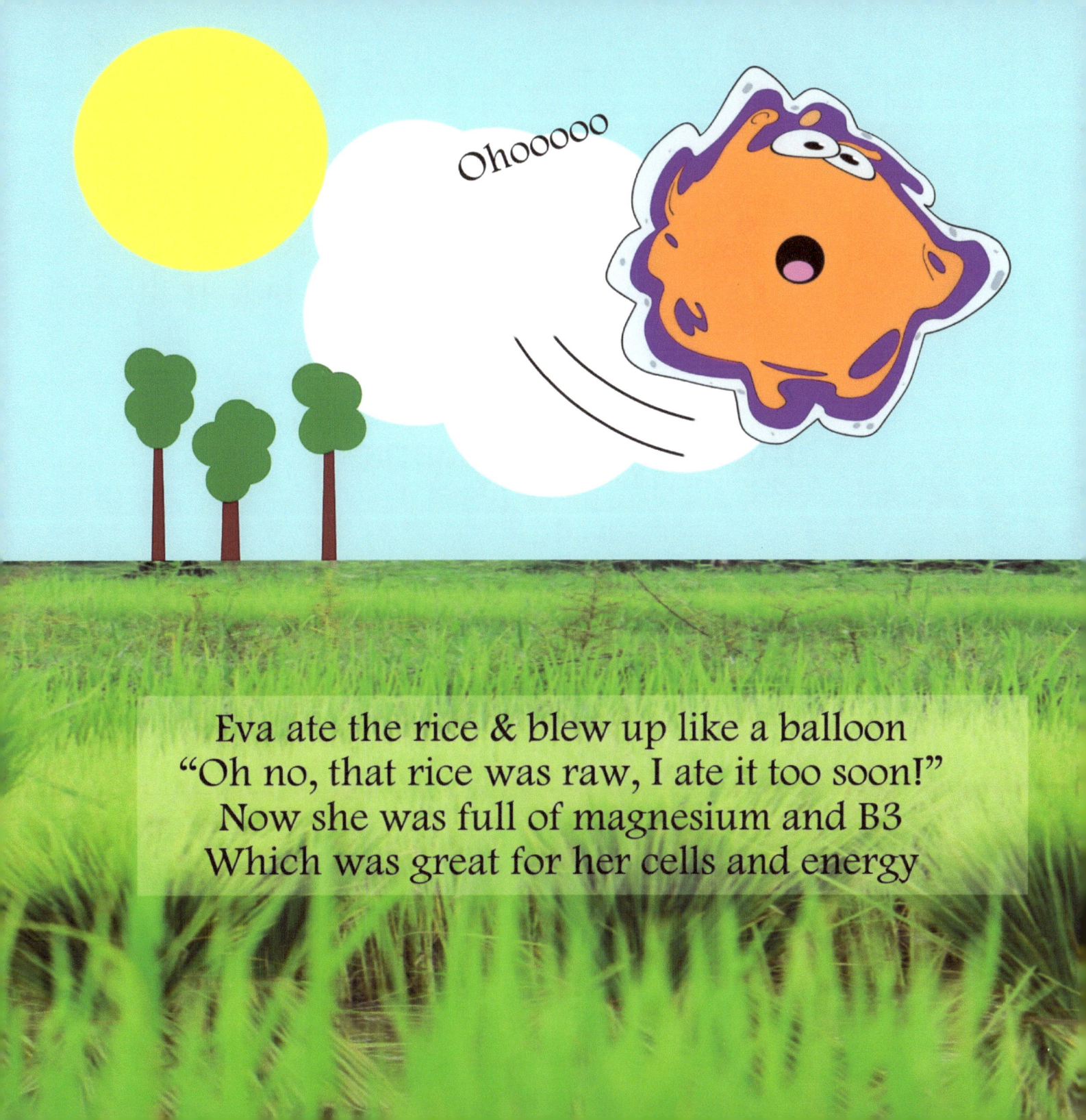

Eva ate the rice & blew up like a balloon
"Oh no, that rice was raw, I ate it too soon!"
Now she was full of magnesium and B3
Which was great for her cells and energy

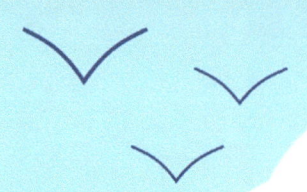

Now Eva was happy and on a roll
She found loads more food, while on her stroll

Enter the Broad Beans

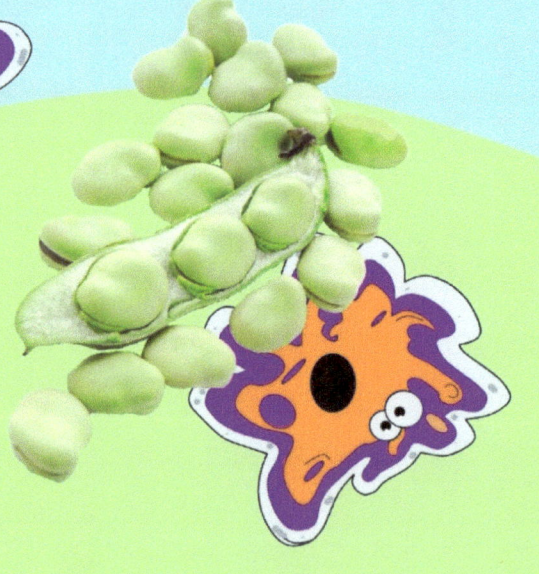

and Baked Beans

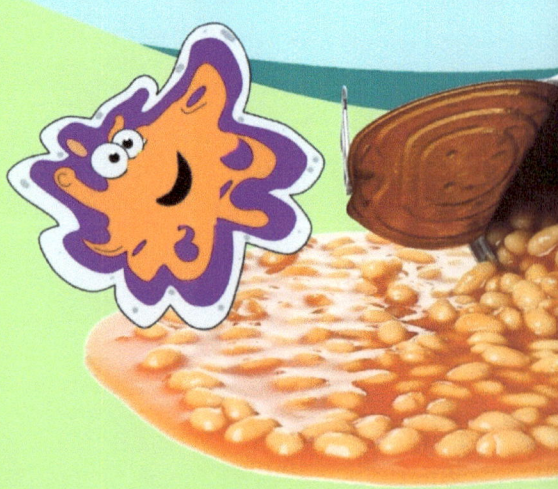

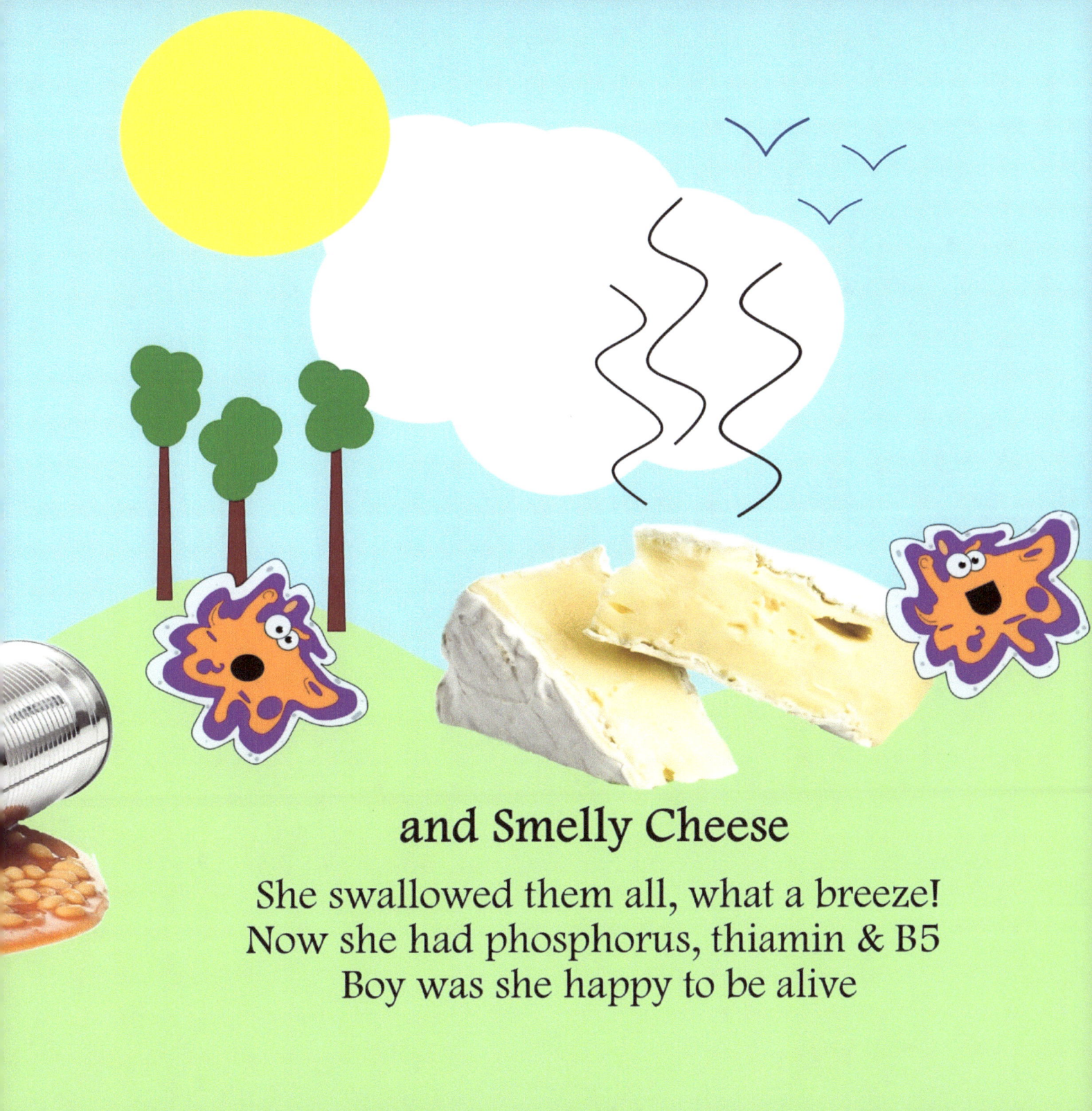

and Smelly Cheese

She swallowed them all, what a breeze!
Now she had phosphorus, thiamin & B5
Boy was she happy to be alive

Eva had just one more food to eat
Before she performed a very great feat
When she saw some fruits, juicy & luscious
Wow, she thought, they look really scrumptious

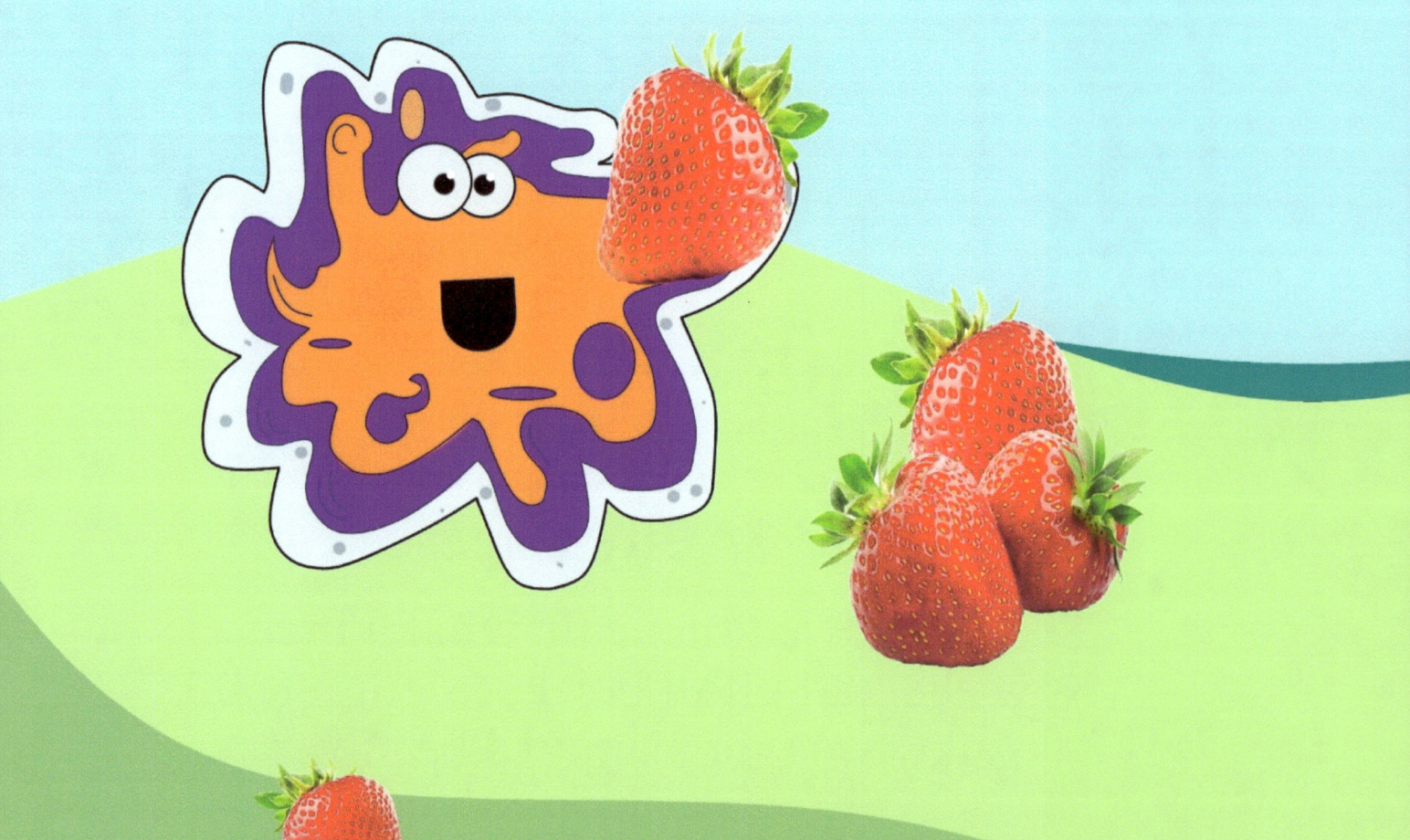

Enter the Strawberries

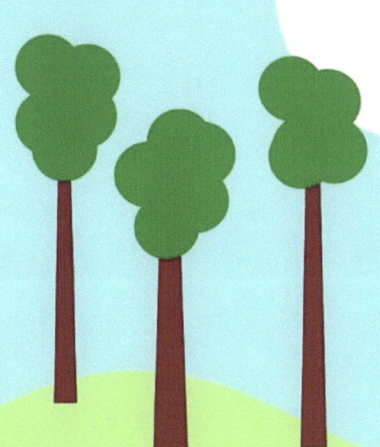

Down they went & with them
Phytochemicals too
Whoa, that's a big word
What do they do?

Well, they protect your cells
To keep you well
And help your DNA
& cells to gel

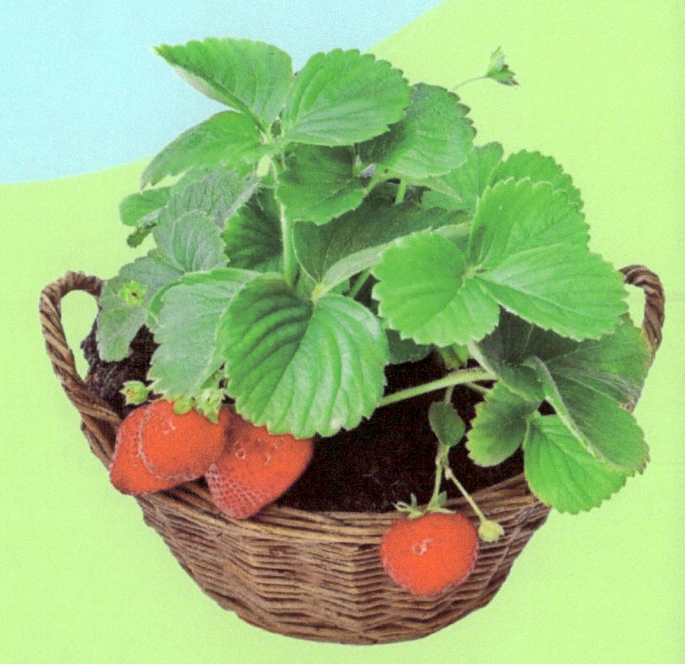

Now Eva had everything she needed
For her first stage of growth, to be completed

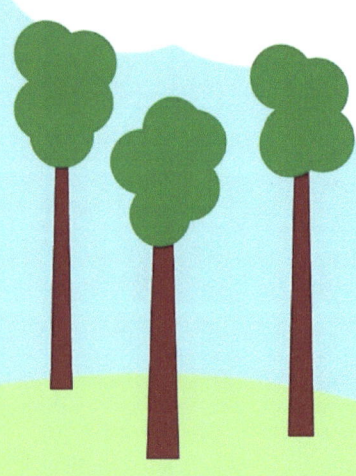

Inside, her cells were changing
Dividing, multiplying, rearranging
But what would happen, she didn't know
Oh my goodness, how would she grow?

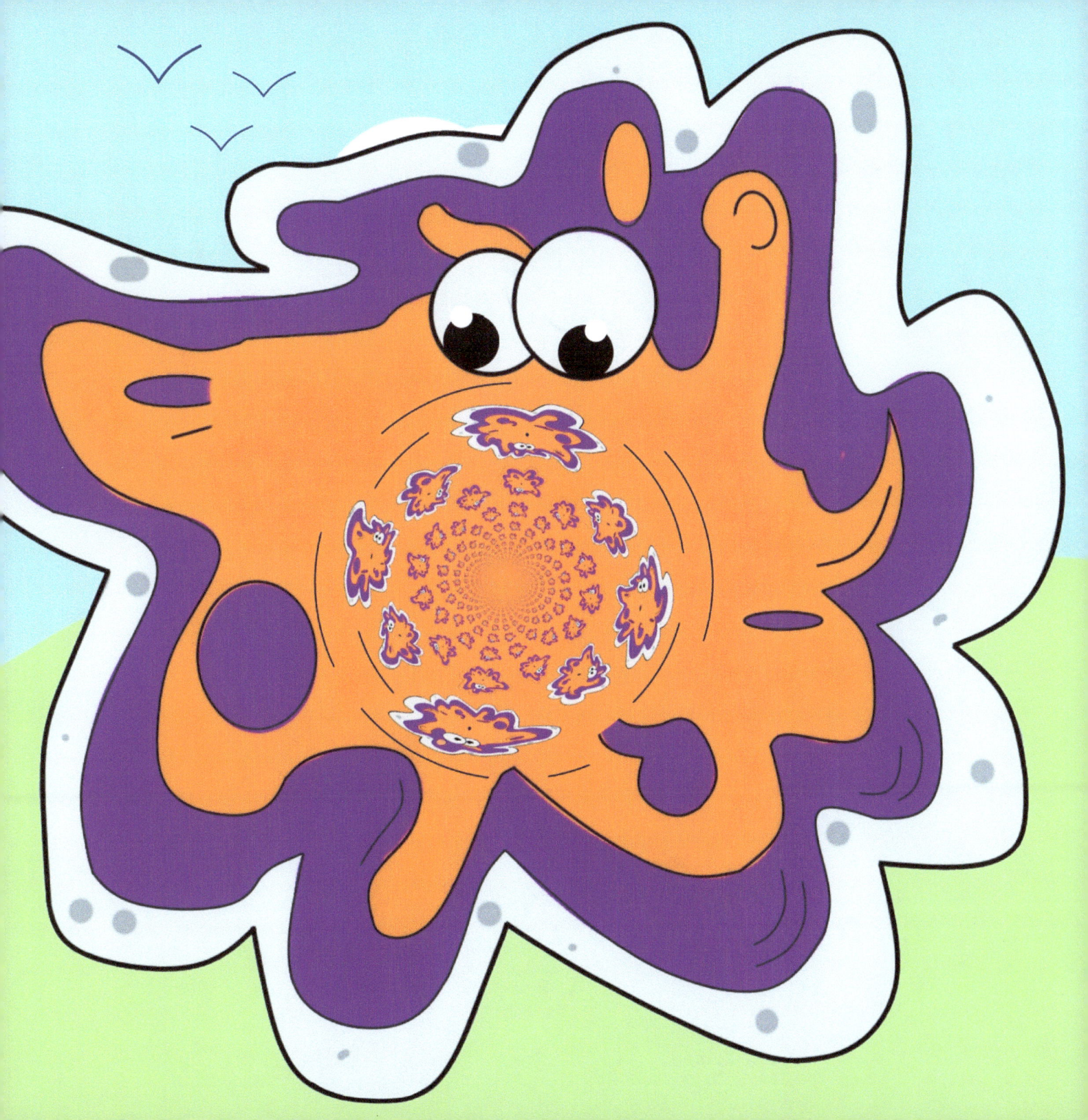

On and on they went
And though it took a while
Her cells had divided
Now she had a face
And a proper smile!

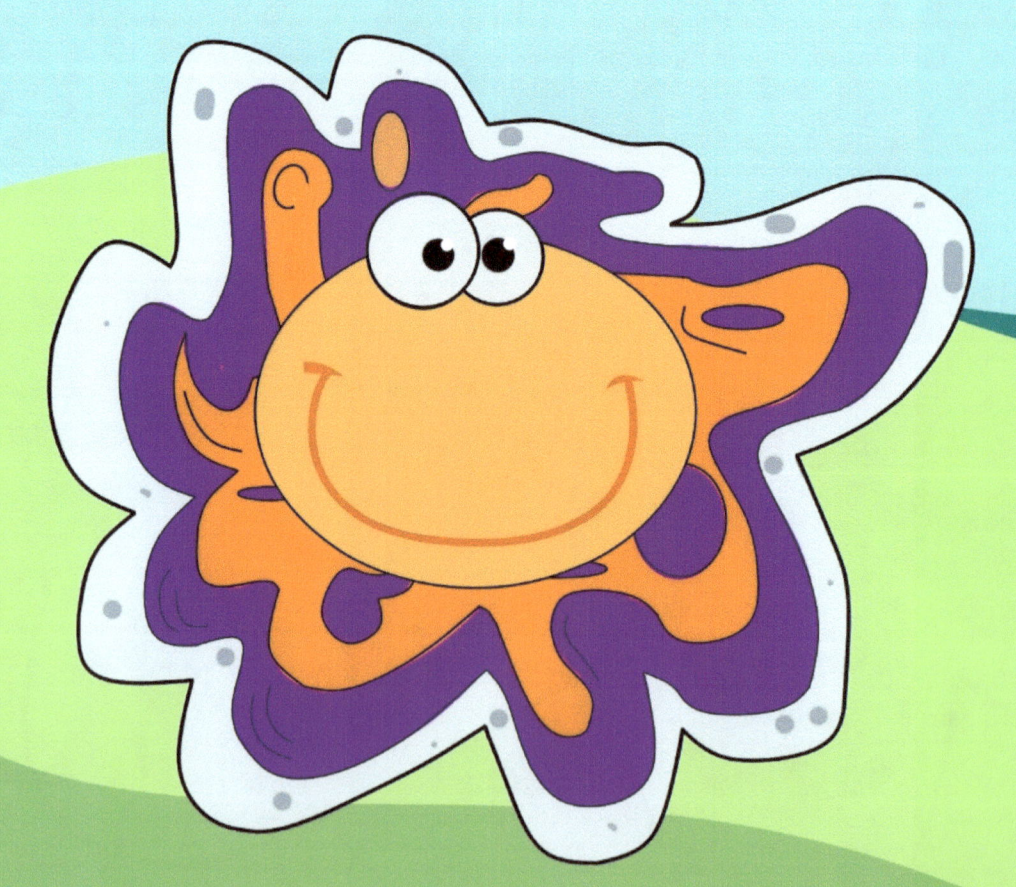

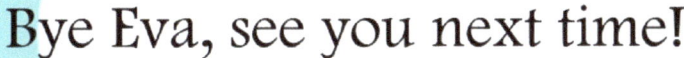

Bye Eva, see you next time!

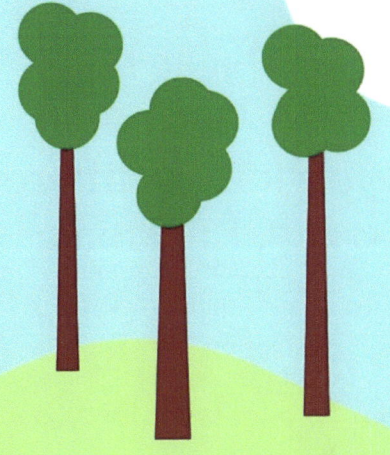

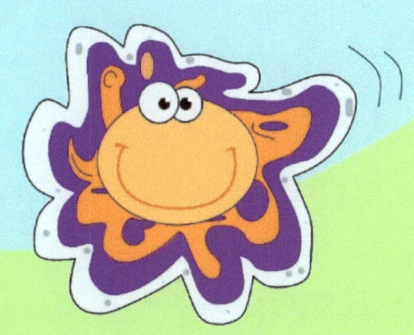

Join Eva on her next adventure
Where she goes to a very
Surprising party

Talking points:

Eva Goes on an Adventure - DNA and Cells

What's an amoeba? - Amoeba's are made of just one cell and look a bit like blobs of jelly.

What's a cell? – A single cell like Eva is the most basic living thing.

People are made up of millions of cells. There are lots of different types of cells (around 210) like those on page 6 & 7, they make you what you are.

What's DNA? – DNA is essential for life. It acts sort of like a computer program and tells your cells what to do.

What are nutrients? – Nutrients are essential substances in foods that your body processes to make energy; to grow, repair and keep your body working smoothly.

All of the nutrients in Eva Goes on an Adventure are essential for healthy DNA and cell replication, but they are also good for a host of other things.

Enter the hazelnut:

Biotin - Vitamin B7
- For the healthy activity of your cells
- It regulates your DNA
- It regulates inflammation
- It protects the development of babies

Enter the Spinach:

Folate - Vitamin B9
- Is essential for DNA creation and repair
- Prevents birth defects
- Lowers the risk of heart disease and cancer
- Regulates inflammation
- Is essential for your brain to function normally

Enter the Eggs:

Vitamin B12
- Is essential for your DNA to duplicate
- Works with folate & vitamin B6 to decrease your risk of heart disease and cancer

Enter the Rice:

Magnesium
- Is essential for creating DNA
- Turns fats and carbs into energy for your cells

Niacin - Vitamin B3
- Keeps your cells talking to each other to keep you healthy
- Is vital for your energy production
- May play a significant role in the prevention of cancer

Enter the broad beans, baked beans and cheese:

Phosphorus
- Is needed by every cell in your body to work normally
- Is critical in creating your energy
- Maintains the chemical balance of your body

Thiamin - Vitamin B1
- Is needed for the creation of DNA,
- Is essential for the creation of energy from your food
- Protects your eyes

Pantothenic acid - Vitamin B5
- Keeps your cells in good order
- Enables your liver to cope with toxins
- Plays a vital role in generating energy from your food

Enter the Strawberries:

Phytochemicals
- The strawberry contains a group of chemicals (known as phytochemicals) that the berry uses to protect itself from disease, and eating strawberries passes on this protection to us
- Phytochemicals provide protection for your DNA and cell replication by keeping your cells communicating clearly with each other

All of these foods have many more fantastic health giving nutrients.
Find out more at **www.checkyourfood.com**

Introducing the subject of nutrition at a young age will allow children to grow up with a healthy understanding of foods and what they do for you.

The companion book to the series, for adults and older children, **The Genius of Ordinary Food** is available on **Amazon**.

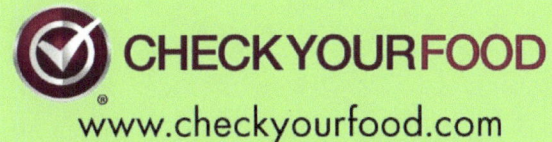

www.checkyourfood.com